This Journal Belongs to...

Published by Meandering Publishing
Copyright 2019 Meandering Publishing

You Are Amazing...
You Got This...
You Can Do Anything!

What makes YOU Amazing?

I love living in my unique female body. It has features that are distinctive and make me who I am.

What is one thing you need to do more of?

I am a strong, confident woman and I will only become stronger.

Write about the best or the worst day of your life:

I choose to release love, happiness, and gratitude into the world today. Life is precious and beautiful and I choose to focus on the positive.

What am I most grateful for this week?

_____
_____
_____
_____
_____
_____
_____
_____
_____
_____
_____
_____
_____
_____
_____

I know I am alive for a reason. Today, I honor my purpose and inspire people around me to do the same.

What are your top five favorite things about yourself?

I will maintain a positive attitude today despite any hurdles that come my way. I have what it takes to succeed.

Who is the one friend you can always rely on?

I am on earth for a reason, and I am committed to living a positive life and being a positive influence on others.

List 10 hobbies and/or activities that bring you joy:

_____
_____
_____
_____
_____
_____
_____
_____
_____
_____
_____
_____
_____
_____
_____
_____
_____
_____
_____
_____

I am in charge of how I feel and today I am choosing happiness.

What is your favorite family tradition? Who started it?

Today might be a rough day, but I won't stop smiling.

Describe your most memorable interaction with a stranger:

I know exactly what I need to do to achieve success, and today I'll start.

Describe your favorite smell in detail:

With every breath out, I release stress from my body.

Write a letter thanking your favorite high school teacher for their impact on your life (bonus: rip out this page and send it to them).

The success of others will not make me jealous. My time will come.

What is your favorite part of your daily routine?

I will say "No" when I don't have the time or inclination to act.

What is one thing you need to let go of today?

My happiness is not dependent on circumstance. Instead, I choose joy.

List 10 things you are looking forward to in the next year:

_____

_____

_____

_____

_____

_____

_____

_____

_____

_____

_____

_____

_____

_____

_____

_____

_____

_____

_____

_____

I trust today not to random chance, but to my own intuition and judgement.

What is the weirdest thing you and a friend have done together?

I am loved. I am wanted. I am perfect just as I am.

What is the #1 lesson your job is teaching you right now?

My presence is a gift to others.

If I could talk to my teenage self, the one thing I would say is?

_____
_____
_____
_____
_____
_____
_____
_____
_____
_____
_____
_____
_____
_____
_____
_____
_____

I will do my best and forget the rest.

Make a list of 30 things that make you smile. :)

My mind, body, and soul are are fit and strong.

What is my strongest character quality?

Fear, hate, and sadness will not have a hold on my life today.

Is there anyone I could begin mentoring?

_____
_____
_____
_____
_____
_____
_____
_____
_____
_____
_____
_____
_____
_____
_____
_____
_____
_____

When my need is strong enough, I will find a way.

Describe your perfect day. Next, what do you need to do in the next year to make that day happen?

I will see the good in every situation.

What do you love most about life?

_____
_____
_____
_____
_____
_____
_____
_____
_____
_____
_____
_____
_____
_____
_____
_____

Life will not happen to me. I won't live with regrets. Today I seize my destiny and forge ahead.

What's surprised you the most about your life or life in general?

I will finish all of my overdue tasks and reduce the overwhelm in my life.

What gives me the most energy?

I am not afraid of change, instead, I embrace it and use it to grow stronger.

What are your top five unanswered questions?

_____
_____
_____
_____
_____
_____
_____
_____
_____
_____
_____
_____
_____
_____
_____
_____
_____
_____
_____
_____
_____

Today I smile.

I feel happiest in my skin when:

Challenges are opportunities to prove to myself that I can do anything I set my mind to.

I'd like to thank my mother for?

Calm is my modus operandi.

I'd to thank my Dad for?

Today I will carpe lucem (seize the light).

Make a list of everything you'd like to say no to:

_____
_____
_____
_____
_____
_____
_____
_____
_____
_____
_____
_____
_____
_____
_____
_____
_____
_____

My time has come. I am powerful, strong, happy, and content with my life.

Make a list of everything you'd like to say yes to:

_____
_____
_____
_____
_____
_____
_____
_____
_____
_____
_____
_____
_____
_____
_____
_____
_____
_____
_____

I end this journal with powerful action steps towards a life changed.

I would like to thank myself for?

_____

_____

_____

_____

_____

_____

_____

_____

_____

_____

_____

_____

_____

_____

_____

_____

Made in the USA
Columbia, SC
30 March 2019